BODYBUILDING FOR BEGINNERS

The most palatable approach to
Building the body of your dreams

Andrew Schwarzenegger

Table of Contents

CHAPTER ONE

Introduction to Bodybuilding

Bodybuilding is a form of physical exercise and body modification that involves the development of skeletal muscle through resistance training, typically using weights. The primary goal of bodybuilding is to sculpt and enhance one's physique, emphasizing muscle size, symmetry, and definition. Bodybuilders often engage in a combination of strength training, cardiovascular exercise, and nutrition to achieve their desired results.

Setting Fitness Goals

Setting clear and realistic fitness goals is crucial for a successful bodybuilding journey. Goals provide direction, motivation, and a sense of accomplishment. Whether aiming for muscle growth, fat loss, increased strength, or overall health improvement, establishing specific, measurable, achievable, relevant, and time-bound (SMART) goals is key. Regularly reassess and adjust these goals as you progress.

Understanding Basic Anatomy

A foundational understanding of basic anatomy is essential for effective bodybuilding. Knowing the major muscle groups, their functions, and how they work together is crucial for targeted training. Common muscle groups include chest, back, shoulders, arms, legs, and core. Proper form during exercises helps prevent injuries and ensures that muscles are worked effectively.

Importance of Nutrition

Nutrition plays a pivotal role in bodybuilding. A well-balanced diet provides the necessary nutrients for muscle growth, energy, and recovery. Adequate protein intake is particularly important, as it supports muscle repair and synthesis. Carbohydrates provide energy for workouts, while fats are essential for overall health. Proper hydration is also crucial for optimal performance and recovery.

Introduction to Strength Training

Strength training is a fundamental aspect of bodybuilding. It involves using resistance, such as weights or resistance bands, to build muscle strength and size. Compound exercises, which engage multiple muscle groups, are often favored in strength training routines. Examples include squats, deadlifts, bench presses, and overhead presses. Consistent progression in weight and intensity is key for continuous muscle development.

Rest and Recovery

Rest and recovery are integral components of any bodybuilding program. Muscles need time to repair and grow stronger after intense workouts. Overtraining can lead to fatigue, increased risk of injury, and hindered progress. Adequate sleep, rest days, and proper recovery techniques, such as stretching and foam rolling, contribute to overall well-being and improved performance.

Bodybuilding is a holistic approach to physical fitness that involves goal setting, understanding anatomy, prioritizing nutrition, engaging in strength training, and allowing for proper rest and recovery. A balanced and disciplined approach to these elements will contribute to a successful and sustainable bodybuilding journey.

Basics of Nutrient Intake

Proper nutrient intake is crucial for overall health and plays a significant role in supporting various physiological functions. The three main macronutrients are carbohydrates, proteins, and fats, each serving distinct purposes in the body. Micronutrients, including vitamins and minerals, are also essential for maintaining health.

Building a Balanced Diet

A balanced diet involves consuming a variety of foods that provide the necessary nutrients in appropriate proportions. This includes a mix of fruits, vegetables, whole grains, lean proteins, and healthy fats. The goal is to ensure an adequate intake of essential nutrients while avoiding excessive amounts of unhealthy or processed foods.

Portion control is key to maintaining a healthy weight and preventing overconsumption of calories.

Importance of Protein

Protein is a critical macronutrient that plays a vital role in various bodily functions. It is essential for the repair and growth of tissues, making it particularly important for individuals engaged in physical activities like bodybuilding. Good sources of protein include lean meats, poultry, fish, dairy products, eggs, legumes, and plant-based sources like tofu and quinoa. Adequate protein intake supports muscle development, immune function, and the synthesis of enzymes and hormones.

Carbohydrates and Energy

Carbohydrates are the body's primary source of energy. They are classified into simple carbohydrates (sugars) and complex carbohydrates (starches and fibers). Whole grains, fruits, vegetables, and legumes are excellent sources of complex carbohydrates, providing sustained energy and essential nutrients. Athletes, including bodybuilders, often rely on carbohydrates to fuel workouts and replenish glycogen stores.

Essential Fats

Fats are essential for overall health and are involved in various physiological processes, including hormone production, absorption of fat-soluble vitamins, and cell structure. Healthy fats include monounsaturated fats and polyunsaturated fats, which are found in sources like avocados, nuts, seeds, and fatty fish. It's important to moderate saturated and trans fats found in processed and fried foods, as excessive intake can contribute to cardiovascular issues.

Building a balanced diet involves understanding the role of macronutrients (carbohydrates, proteins, and fats) and incorporating a variety of nutrient-dense foods into daily meals. Proper nutrient intake supports overall health, energy levels, and specific fitness goals, making it an integral part of any bodybuilding or fitness journey.

CHAPTER TWO

Introduction to Workout Splits

Workout splits refer to how you organize your training sessions throughout the week, focusing on different muscle groups or movement patterns during each session. The choice of workout split depends on individual goals, preferences, and training experience. Common workout splits include full-body workouts, targeted muscle group training, and variations that focus on specific areas of the body.

Full-Body Workouts

Full-body workouts involve training all major muscle groups in a single session. This approach is suitable for beginners or individuals with limited time for training. Full-body workouts typically include compound exercises that engage multiple muscle groups simultaneously, promoting overall strength and muscle development. These workouts are often performed two to three times per week.

Targeted Muscle Group Training

Targeted muscle group training involves dedicating specific training sessions to particular muscle groups. Common splits include training different muscle groups on separate days, such as chest and triceps, back and biceps, and legs. This approach allows for more focused work on individual muscle groups, enabling greater volume and intensity for each targeted area.

Importance of Progressive Overload

Progressive overload is a fundamental principle in strength training and bodybuilding. It involves gradually increasing the demands placed on the muscles to stimulate growth and adaptation. This can be achieved by progressively increasing weight, reps, or intensity over time. Without progressive overload, the body may not experience the necessary stimulus for continued improvement.

Cardiovascular Exercise for Health

While bodybuilding often emphasizes resistance training,

cardiovascular exercise is crucial for overall health and fitness. Cardio workouts, such as running, cycling, or swimming, enhance cardiovascular health, improve endurance, and aid in fat loss. Incorporating a mix of aerobic and anaerobic activities can contribute to a well-rounded fitness routine.

Flexibility and Mobility

Flexibility and mobility are often overlooked but essential components of a comprehensive fitness program. Stretching and mobility exercises help maintain joint health, improve range of motion, and reduce the risk of injuries. Incorporating dynamic stretches, static stretches, and mobility drills can enhance overall flexibility and joint function.

Effective workout planning involves choosing an appropriate workout split, whether it's full-body workouts or targeted muscle group training. Progressive overload is key to stimulating muscle growth and strength improvement. Balancing resistance training with cardiovascular exercise, flexibility, and mobility work contributes to a holistic approach to fitness and well-being.

Basics of Weightlifting

Weightlifting is a form of strength training that involves lifting weights to build muscle strength, power, and endurance. It is a fundamental component of many fitness programs and sports training. Understanding the basics of weightlifting is crucial for safe and effective workouts.

Proper Form and Technique

Proper form and technique are paramount in weightlifting to prevent injuries and maximize effectiveness. Each exercise has a specific movement pattern, and maintaining correct form ensures that the targeted muscles are engaged while minimizing stress on joints. Beginners should start with lighter weights and focus on mastering proper technique before progressing to heavier loads.

Common Strength Training Exercises

There are several common strength training exercises that target major muscle groups:

Squats: Work the muscles in the lower body, particularly the quadriceps, hamstrings, and glutes.

Deadlifts: Engage the muscles in the back, hips, and legs, emphasizing the posterior chain.

Bench Press: Targets the chest, shoulders, and triceps.

Overhead Press (Shoulder Press): Focuses on the shoulders and triceps.

Rows: Strengthen the muscles in the upper back.

Pull-Ups/Chin-Ups: Work the muscles in the back and arms.

Lunges: Engage the lower body muscles and improve balance.

Reps, Sets, and Rest Periods

Understanding the concepts of reps, sets, and rest periods is crucial for designing an effective weightlifting program. A repetition (rep) is one complete movement of an exercise, while a set is a specific number of consecutive reps. The number of sets and reps, as well as the rest periods between sets, can be manipulated to achieve different training goals. For example, lower reps with heavier weights focus on strength, while higher reps with lighter weights target muscle endurance.

Avoiding Common Mistakes

To ensure a safe and effective weightlifting routine, it's important to avoid common mistakes:

Lifting too much weight: Gradually progress to heavier weights to avoid injuries.

Poor form: Maintain proper form throughout each repetition to prevent injuries and maximize results.

Skipping warm-up: Warm up before lifting weights to increase blood flow, flexibility, and reduce the risk of injury.

Neglecting rest and recovery: Allow sufficient time for rest and recovery to avoid overtraining and promote muscle growth.

Incorporating Variations for Progress

Incorporating variations of exercises is essential for ongoing progress. Changing grips, foot positions, or using different equipment can target muscles from different angles and prevent plateaus. Periodically adjusting the training routine also keeps workouts challenging and engaging.

Weightlifting is a powerful tool for building strength and muscle mass. Focusing on proper form, incorporating common strength training exercises, understanding reps, sets, and rest periods, avoiding common mistakes, and incorporating variations are key elements to a successful and sustainable weightlifting program.

CHAPTER THREE

Introduction to Gym Equipment

Gym equipment plays a crucial role in various fitness routines, providing options for resistance training, cardiovascular exercise, and flexibility training. Understanding the different types of equipment available can help individuals design effective and diverse workout programs.

Dumbbells and Barbells

Dumbbells and barbells are versatile free weights commonly used for strength training. They allow for a wide range of exercises targeting different muscle groups. Dumbbells are handheld weights used for unilateral exercises, while barbells are long bars with weights on each end, often used for compound movements like squats and deadlifts. They provide stability challenges and engage stabilizer muscles, promoting overall strength development.

Weight Machines

Weight machines are stationary equipment with predefined movement patterns and resistance. They are user-friendly, making them suitable for beginners. Weight machines often target specific muscle groups and provide a guided range of motion. They are beneficial for isolating muscles and can be a valuable addition to a well-rounded workout routine.

Resistance Bands

Resistance bands are elastic bands that provide resistance during exercises. They come in various resistance levels and can be used for both upper and lower body workouts. Resistance bands are portable, affordable, and effective for adding resistance to bodyweight exercises or enhancing traditional weightlifting movements. They are particularly useful for improving strength, stability, and flexibility.

Bodyweight Exercises

Bodyweight exercises utilize the individual's own body weight as resistance. Examples include push-ups, squats, lunges, and planks. Bodyweight exercises are effective for building strength, flexibility, and endurance. They are versatile, require minimal equipment, and can be adapted to various fitness levels.

Choosing the Right Equipment for Your Goals

Selecting the right equipment for your fitness goals depends on individual preferences, fitness levels, and objectives. If the goal is to build muscle mass, free weights like dumbbells and barbells may be preferred. Those aiming for convenience and ease of use may opt for weight machines. Resistance bands are excellent for individuals looking for a portable and versatile option. Bodyweight exercises are suitable for those who prefer minimal equipment or are new to fitness.

Understanding the characteristics and benefits of different gym equipment allows individuals to create diverse and effective workout routines. The right combination of equipment can cater to specific fitness goals, whether it be strength training, cardiovascular fitness, or overall well-being.

Mental Health and Fitness

Mental health is closely interconnected with physical fitness. Regular exercise has been shown to positively impact mood, reduce stress, and contribute to overall well-being. Physical activity stimulates the release of endorphins, the body's natural mood lifters. Incorporating exercise into your routine can enhance mental clarity, improve sleep, and contribute to a positive mindset.

Creating a Consistent Routine

Creating a consistent fitness routine is crucial for long-term success. Consistency is key to achieving fitness goals and maintaining overall health. Establishing a regular schedule helps make exercise a habit. Choose a time that fits your lifestyle, whether it's morning, lunchtime, or evening, and find activities you enjoy to make sticking to your routine more enjoyable.

Tracking Progress and Adjustments

Tracking progress is essential for monitoring your fitness journey. Keep a record of your workouts, noting the exercises, sets, and weights used. Track changes in strength, endurance, or body composition over time. Regularly reassess your goals and make adjustments to your workout routine to ensure continued progress. This might involve increasing intensity, changing exercises, or modifying your overall plan.

Injury Prevention and Recovery

Injury prevention and recovery are integral to maintaining a consistent fitness routine. Warm up properly before workouts, use proper form during exercises, and listen to your body. Adequate rest and recovery are equally important; include rest days in your routine, prioritize quality sleep, and incorporate activities like stretching and foam rolling to enhance flexibility and reduce muscle soreness.

Social Support and Accountability

Social support and accountability can significantly impact your fitness journey. Engage in activities with friends, join group classes, or find a workout buddy. Sharing goals with others creates a sense of accountability, motivation, and community. Having a support system can provide encouragement during challenging times and celebrate achievements together.

Transitioning to Intermediate Bodybuilding

Transitioning to intermediate bodybuilding involves progressing from basic to more advanced training techniques. Focus on refining your form, increasing resistance gradually, and incorporating more diverse exercises. Implementing advanced training principles such as drop sets, supersets, and periodization can help stimulate further muscle growth. Pay attention to recovery strategies and ensure a balanced approach to avoid overtraining.

In summary, the connection between mental health and fitness underscores the importance of exercise for overall well-being. Establishing a consistent routine, tracking progress, preventing injuries, and seeking social support contribute to a successful fitness journey. As you progress, transitioning to intermediate bodybuilding involves refining your approach and incorporating more advanced techniques for continued growth and development.

THE END